Intermittent Fasting

How To Transform Your Body Into A Fat-burning
Machine And Shed Pounds

I0105470

*(A Comprehensive Guide For Men To Lose Weight, Increase
Energy, And Balance Hormones)*

Milorad Nussbaumer

TABLE OF CONTENT

Introduction

Intermittent fasting is not a diet, but rather a pattern of eating. Dietary planning is a method for maximizing the nutritional value of food intake. Intermittent fasting does not alter what you eat, but rather when you eat. The objective of intermittent fasting is to lengthen the time between the last meal of one day and the first meal of the next.

According to studies, intermittent fasting aids in weight management and may be capable of reversing certain diseases.

Johns Hopkins neurologist Mark Mattson has studied intermittent fasting for 25 years. According to him, our bodies have evolved to be able to survive without food for an extended period of time, possibly for days. In the prehistoric era, humans were hunters and gatherers before they discovered how to cultivate crops. They evolved to be able to survive and thrive during long periods without food. Therefore, they had to devote a great deal of time and energy to hunting wildlife and gathering nuts and berries.

Due to the fact that animals, including humans, evolved in environments where food was scarce, they have developed numerous adaptations that allow them to perform at a high level, both physically and cognitively, when food-deprived/fasting.

Intermittent fasting (IF) refers to recurrent eating patterns in which individuals go for extended time periods (e.g., 16–48 h) with little or no energy intake, followed by normal eating periods.

In modern society, people frequently consume food three or more times per day. Especially when coupled with a sedentary lifestyle, excessive food consumption and such eating patterns frequently result in metabolic morbidities (insulin resistance, excessive visceral fat deposition, etc.).

Eating more calories and being less active can increase the risk of obesity, type 2 diabetes, cardiovascular disease, and other ailments.

When you practise intermittent fasting, you eat only during the allotted hours. Your body can burn fat if you fast for a specific amount of time each day or eat only one meal a few times per week.

After several hours without food, the body begins to burn fat because it has run out of sugar. Changing metabolism is the term for this process.

Intermittent fasting is effective because it lengthens the time until your body has burned off the calories from your last meal and begins to burn fat.

Autophagy is a process related to fasting that is attracting a great deal of interest due to its possible health benefits. When you are well-nourished, your cells and their components are highly acetylated.

This suggests that acetyl groups are attached to the lysine (amino acid) residues of a number of cellular components, including the "packaging" proteins called histones that neatly encase your DNA within the cell nucleus.

When you are not fasting, your cells activate genes that promote cellular development and proliferation while inhibiting the activity of other genes. There are genes involved in fat metabolism, stress tolerance, and damage repair among these. In fact, intermittent fasting causes a portion of your body fat to be converted into ketone bodies, which appear to stimulate these genes, resulting in decreased inflammation and stress resistance in the brain, for example.

Short-term fasting can induce ketosis, a metabolic state in which the body breaks down fat stores for energy in the absence of sufficient glucose. This leads to the formation of ketone-like compounds. In addition to consuming fewer calories overall, this can result in weight loss.

In this state, the body starts to digest and burn fat.

A portion of this fat is used by the liver to produce ketone bodies (ketones). When glucose is not readily available, the cells of the heart, skeletal muscle, and brain can utilise the two primary ketones, acetoacetate and -hydroxybutyrate (BHB).

During intermittent fasting, the liver produces ketone bodies, which partially replace glucose as the brain and other organs' energy source. When ketones are metabolised, they generate fewer inflammatory byproducts than glucose and can even stimulate the production of the brain growth factor BDNF! This ketone utilisation by the brain is one of the reasons why intermittent fasting is frequently claimed to promote mental clarity and positive mood! In addition, it has been demonstrated that ketones can reduce inflammation in a variety of cell types and reduce cellular damage and apoptosis in neurons.

In addition, fasting has an effect on the metabolic functions of the body, which may help to improve blood sugar control, reduce inflammation, and enhance the body's ability to respond to physical stress. According to a number of studies, this may assist with inflammatory diseases such as multiple sclerosis, asthma, and arthritis.

Chapter 1: What Is Intermittent Fasting?

Intermittent fasting is currently one of the most popular health and fitness trends on the planet. People use it to lose weight, improve their health, and simplify their lives.

Numerous studies indicate that it can have profound effects on your body and brain, and may even improve your quality of life.

Intermittent fasting may be a fascinating topic to study, but it is easy to become confused when researching it. There is so much freely available information on intermittent fasting that beginners and people over the age of 50 may have difficulty getting started. To help people understand intermittent fasting and all of its benefits, I have written a fantastic book about this nutritional phenomenon.

Key Foods and Nutrients for a Healthy Fasting Program:

If you pay attention to these foods, you will likely achieve successful fasting results. Omega-3 fatty acids - the benefits of cardiovascular protection and anti-obesity properties of omega fatty acids are well documented in scientific literature. Eating fatty fish or taking a high-quality fish oil supplement is an excellent way to provide your brain with the proper nutrients to combat caloric restriction side effects.

Vitamins C and D - regarding fish, fasting typically results in low levels of these vitamins, so it is essential to include them in your fasting diet. Fish is an excellent source of vitamin D, and berries are an excellent source of vitamin C. Resveratrol is also very protective and anti-inflammatory.

During fasting, the levels of calcium, chromium, sodium, and potassium tend to drop significantly. Eggs are calcium-rich, nutritious, and a low-calorie way to satisfy hunger. Nuts are an excellent snack during fasting because they are densely packed with chromium, potassium, and other essential nutrients, and they may also send signals to the brain that prevent hunger. Again, berries are a potent weapon in the nutritional arsenal.

Probiotics - one irritating effect of fasting is that your microbiome expresses its displeasure at being hungry, which can contribute to stomach discomfort, constipation, and other problems. Yogurt and kefir are probiotic-rich foods that can alleviate these issues and keep your stomach happy for very few calories. Fermented cabbage, such as kimchi or sauerkraut, is another health-destroying food that will accomplish the task and add fibre and nutrients to the mixture.

Additionally, AMPK-rich foods stimulate the metabolism, which is crucial to the entire process. We want our bodies to shift into fat-burning survival mode, which is the basis of the fasting benefits. Berries, particularly maqui berries, are the most potent metabolic stimulants by weight. These incredible foods pack a tremendous nutritional punch for their calories. Berry consumption during fasting not only nourishes AMPK for enhanced metabolic function, but also provides a full spectrum of essential vitamins and minerals. During fasting, if you could only consume one meal, berries may be the best option.

Curcumin is quite effective as an anti-inflammatory during the fasting phase, promotes weight loss, and improves the body's stress tolerance, which is crucial during intermittent fasting. Curcumin and resveratrol function similarly and are excellent fasting supplements.

Everyone has different nutritional needs, so this is a general and by no means exhaustive guide. Before beginning a fasting programme, you may wish to obtain a baseline blood test, and you should consult your primary care physician to avoid complications. The premise of this article is that it may be advantageous to restrict your body's food intake at times, but you must be even more careful about what you consume during the process. Observe these few essential requirements. You will notice a pattern: immune and metabolic boosters, anti-inflammatory foods, preventative meals, and nutrients. Concentrate on them to promote vitality and longevity.

Chapter 2: Exercise Suggestions During An Intermittent Fast

Take your time. Try increasing the intensity of your workouts gradually as your body adjusts to your new diet, as there is no single strategy that will work for everyone. "An hour of exercise in the morning will be too much for those who are accustomed to eating beforehand." However, if you only exercise for 15 or 20 minutes during the transition, you may be able to get away with it.

Consider your preferred exercise time of day. If you only exercise before 8 a.m., you may need to adjust your eating schedule so you can eat immediately after a cardio session. If you enjoy working out in the late afternoon, lifting weights is the optimal activity. You may perform low-intensity workouts at any time of day.

Your dining window should be spacious. If you enjoy morning runs as much as your friend does, a 12-to-8-hour eating window will not be as effective for you. You may need to alter your eating schedule to 9 a.m. to 5 p.m. in order to consume a protein drink after a workout.

Hydrate. You should not skimp on water simply because you have not eaten in a while. A person who practises intermittent fasting must stay hydrated if they wish to engage in fasted exercise. Each day, consume at least 72 ounces of water, or more if you perspire heavily.

Employ electrolytes. Natural sports drinks or other low-calorie solutions, such as coconut water, can replenish electrolytes in your body without breaking your fast.

Try out different exercises. A combination of strength training and cardiovascular exercise will help you burn fat and build muscle. Additionally, you can use this to assist with your IF schedule. On days you can exercise in the morning, cardio should be your primary focus; on days you must exercise in the evening, strength training should be your best friend. When you are extremely exhausted, skip your workout and try yoga or Pilates instead.

Be conscious of your body. The best exercise regimen for you is one that leaves you feeling energised and strong, as opposed to exhausted. What will make us feel better is what our bodies indicate is best for us. Attend this spin class four times per week, but refrain from exerting yourself to the point of exhaustion.

To help your body become accustomed to exercising while fasting, be careful to ease into your selected exercises, drink plenty of water, be flexible with your eating window, and pay close attention to your body at all times.

Chapter 3: Boosts Vitality And Mental Clarity

In addition to promoting rapid weight loss, intermittent fasting can boost energy levels and mental clarity. In one study, intermittent fasting was shown to improve memory and brain function in mice, while in another, it may improve mood and reduce depressive symptoms.

Fasting provides a break for the digestive system and allows the body to redirect its energy to other functions, resulting in increased energy.

As the body is able to redirect its energy to brain function rather than digestion, it can also result in enhanced concentration and mental clarity.

Effectively improves fat-burning process

In addition to promoting rapid weight loss, intermittent fasting can also increase fat oxidation. One study revealed that intermittent fasting increased levels of human growth hormone, which aids in fat burning and muscle building. During fasting, the body uses stored energy (fat) as fuel, as opposed to continuously supplying energy through food consumption. This can result in a reduction in total body fat.

In addition, intermittent fasting can increase insulin sensitivity, which helps the body burn fat for energy rather than store it.

Chapter 4: The Most Effective Approach To Intermittent Fasting

You have received sufficient information and are prepared to enter the wonderful world of IF. When are you permitted to eat? "The easiest method is to skip breakfast and drink coffee or tea instead," explains Zane. If you want to lose weight, eat a low-carb lunch and dinner. After the fasting window expires, the first meal of the day is consumed, meaning that all meals are consumed within a six- to eight-hour window. "It's a situation of give and take." Ensure that it fits your schedule. If the duration is six hours, that's fantastic. Zane adds, "Don't beat yourself up if it must be nine one day."

The beauty of IF is that there is no right or wrong approach. It is a tool you can use to improve your health in whatever way is most effective for you. Here are some suggestions for an effective intermittent fasting schedule:

After dinner, you should refrain from eating (8:00 PM)

Skipping breakfast and consuming a cup of black coffee or tea until noon.

A low-carb meal can assist in breaking the fast.

If you must snack, choose something light.

Before resuming your fast, have a hearty supper.

Try extending your fast to 1:00, 2:00, or 3:00 a.m. once you've gotten used to the pattern of intermittent fasting.

Step 6: Involve yourself in the dinnertime community

There is a reason why the majority of people choose to skip breakfast over dinner. The nature of your evening meals is social and interpersonal. This has been the case for millennia! You use dinner to decompress from the day, reconcile with family, and mark the passing of another day. You need not miss out on such a rewarding opportunity. Instead, develop mindfulness while you are eating. You will appreciate every bite of dinner much more than if you had nibbled all day. Zane observes with his clients that the most effective method of fasting is to maintain dinner as the primary meal.

Step 7: Consume with Purpose

When it comes to intermittent fasting, you must determine when to consume food. However, what should you consume after opening your mouth? There is no universal solution; everything depends on your goals.

When attempting to Lose Weight.

If you are trying to lose weight, it is recommended that you reduce your consumption of carbohydrates and sugar. Make it as easy as possible by planning each day's meal to break the fast in advance. Preparing a satiating, low-carb lunch can prevent you from making hasty decisions. Dinner should consist of a lean protein and a vegetable, though healthy carbohydrates and fats are also acceptable. Remember that you are rewarding yourself with nutritious and delicious meals, not punishing yourself!

If weight loss is not your primary objective.

Focus on consuming actual foods if you are fasting for the sake of your health and longevity. If it was not food one hundred years ago, it is not food today! Avoid packaged, processed foods and read labels in order to avoid the unseen trap of added sugars. It is essential to consume a diet rich in healthy fats, proteins, and fruits and vegetables. If you consume these actual meals, you will immediately reduce your consumption of those sneaky carbohydrates.

Attempt a 24-hour fast once per week.

Do not worry excessively about the 24-hour fast. After becoming accustomed to intermittent fasting, switching to a once-weekly 24-hour fast is not such a big deal. The best time to begin a 24-hour fast is after dinner. Instead of breaking your fast with lunch at 1:00 p.m., wait a few hours and celebrate with supper. One day of fasting per week, the first meal after a 24-hour fast, is extremely satisfying. It is unlike any other thing. To disregard the fat-burning and metabolic benefits of a 24-hour reset.

Step 9: Avoid Cheat Days While Intermittent Fasting

A cheat day is equivalent to a binge day for the majority of people, except that the effects of the binge last longer than 24 hours. It may take three or four days to recover from the effects of a cheat day, rein in your desires, regain your energy and focus, and get back on track. " Why sabotage your weight-loss efforts with a large pizza or stack of pancakes if you're trying to reach your goal efficiently? During an IF cheat day, an increase of 1,500 calories from junk food will send you in the opposite direction of your goals. On the other hand, an indulgence is a different matter. A slice of pie or a few cookies may help you scratch an urge before it develops into a rash that causes you to become stranded.

Chapter 5: Intermittent Fasting For Women

If you are a woman over the age of 50 and do not know how to lose weight, we have the answer for you. We provide you with a diet based on how many calories you should consume based on your age.

It is advised to consume approximately 1,500 calories per day. However, sedentary women are recommended to consume 1,200 calories per day. Remember that lack of physical activity greatly increases the likelihood of gaining weight.

The areas where fat concentration is greatest are the hips, legs, and abdomen. Significantly affect the body are hormonal fluctuations. For this reason, women of this age have a slower metabolism, which increases the likelihood of weight gain.

In general, the required diet consists of:

Fruits, vegetables, and legumes. The best protein sources are those that are low in fat, such as fish, chicken, turkey, and nuts.

You should consume fat sparingly if it comes from a healthy source, such as olive oil.

To maintain healthy bones, it is necessary to consume at least 1,200 mg of calcium per day. You can consume it through food or as a supplement.

Principal Micronutrient Sources

Regarding dairy products, it is recommended to consume 1- 2 glasses of skim milk or yoghurt per day. 1 cup of yoghurt has roughly the same amount of calcium as 1 cup of milk.

It is also recommended to consume roughly 50 grammes of fresh cheese.

Vitamin D is also required for calcium metabolism, and women over the age of 70 are advised to consume 800 IU per day. In addition to sunlight, certain foods, such as:

Egg yolks

The cheddar

Supplemented dairy products

Ask your physician if a vitamin D supplement would be beneficial.

In addition, it is recommended to consume 2 12 cups of vegetables per day. More variety is preferable. For the digestive organs to function properly and to avoid constipation, older women should consume a diet high in fibre.

Diets low in carbohydrates and high in protein are not recommended for elderly women because they can cause metabolic issues.

It is best to consume predominantly polyunsaturated and monounsaturated fats, such as those found in olive oil. Although you should not consume more than 5–6 tablespoons of oil per day.

Physical activity helps burn the calories consumed, thereby preventing weight gain. This does not imply that senior citizens must join a gym or run a marathon.

5 WEIGHT LOSS AND PERIODICAL FASTING

Implementing intermittent fasting can help you cut calories and shed pounds.

Intermittent fasting is most effective for weight loss due to its capacity to reduce caloric intake. During the fasting periods, all protocols require abstaining from food. You will not consume as many calories unless you eat significantly more at each meal to make up the difference.

A 2014 study discovered that 3–24 weeks of intermittent fasting decreased body weight by 3–8%. (22). Depending on the rate of weight loss, intermittent fasting may result in weekly weight loss between 0.55 and 1.65 pounds (0.25-0.75 kg).

In addition, people's waist circumference decreased by 4-7%, indicating that they lost abdominal fat. These results demonstrate that intermittent fasting can be beneficial. Even though intermittent fasting typically does not require calorie counting, the majority of weight loss is mediated by a reduction in calorie intake.

Studies comparing intermittent fasting and continuous calorie restriction reveal no difference in weight loss when caloric intake is equalised between groups.

Intermittent fasting may help you maintain muscle mass while dieting.

When you diet, your body tends to lose both fat and muscle, which is one of the worst side effects.

Intermittent fasting may help you maintain muscle mass while losing weight, according to some research.

According to a review of the scientific literature, intermittent calorie restriction results in the same amount of weight loss as continuous calorie restriction, but with significantly less muscle mass loss.

In the studies on calorie restriction, muscle mass accounted for 25% of the weight loss, as opposed to only 10% in the studies on intermittent calorie restriction. Consider the results with a grain of salt due to the limitations of the studies. No additional contemporary research has been discovered.

Does intermittent fasting make healthy eating easier?

Simplicity is one of the primary benefits of intermittent fasting for many individuals. Most intermittent fasting regimens only require you to keep track of time, as opposed to calories. The optimal diet for you is one that you can adhere to long-term. If intermittent fasting helps you maintain a healthy diet, it will have long-term health and weight maintenance advantages.

Chapter 6: A Lifestyle That Involves Intermittent Fasting Is Not A Religion.

As intermittent fasting is more than just another diet, it must be practised on a consistent basis for its benefits to be realised. Once you've lost the excess weight, you won't want to stop doing it; rather, you'll want to continue doing it. Intermittent fasting not only makes it easier to maintain a healthy weight, but it also provides an abundance of additional health benefits, as described in the chapter on why you should consider fasting. If you've ever visited Augusta, Georgia during the Masters Golf Tournament, when pollen levels are at their peak, you know it's not uncommon to see yellow pollen drifting through the streets. As an example, my inflammation has decreased to the point where I no longer require daily allergy medication. I experimented with intermittent fasting from 2009 to 2014, but I was never able to convince myself that it was something I wanted or could do permanently. I came to believe that dieting only lasted as long as necessary to achieve the desired weight loss, after which the weight was mysteriously maintained forever and ever, amen. After realising that there was no true finish line and that weight maintenance required some degree of adaptation for the rest of my life, I realised that intermittent fasting was the ONLY way I could envision living my life permanently. After selecting an intermittent fasting plan, you will need to determine how to make it work for you. There is nothing wrong with employing multiple strategies. Check out the examples I've provided in the book, as well as the books I've listed in the Annotated Bibliography. Each of these books contains more information regarding the tactics than I have provided.

Why then do I assert that intermittent fasting is a lifestyle and not a religion? I want you to be able to forgive yourself for being hindered by life. It is acceptable for you to take a day off to enjoy your life. You will need to convert your eating window into a revolving door while on vacation or a holiday. Believe me, I also do it. For intermittent fasting to be effective, daily perfection is not required.

Regardless of the intermittent fasting method you employ, please note the following sentence: you DO NOT need to be perfect. You do not have to feel bad about your failures or like a failure if you take a day off.

The most important aspect is your lifestyle. LIVING. Despite having the most noble intentions, life is messy and imperfect. We both occasionally feast and fast. Hunger is not a sign of weakness; it merely indicates that you are human.

Let me describe a few instances from this year in which I have demonstrated this lifestyle. This summer I participated in TWO cruises. The first was a five-day trip I took with my husband to celebrate our 25th wedding anniversary. The following week, my college best friends and I embarked on a 4-day cruise. What is the cruise industry's reputation? You would be correct in saying "FOOD." I did not fast while on the cruise ship, as you might have anticipated. Even though I frequently skipped breakfast and didn't start eating until midday, I made it a point to consume at least two substantial meals per day, in addition to afternoon (or late-night) buffet trips. Upon disembarking the ship, especially on the second voyage, I had a typical food baby.

After that, I was hesitant to consume a full meal.

I no longer weigh myself, so I am unaware of how my weight has changed as a result of all that eating. I recall that my clothing was tight when I left the second ship, but a week later I felt normal again. My body adjusted, and I immediately resumed my fasting diet as if the excursions had never occurred. Once I returned home, I did not feel remorse or the need to make amends.

This year, I enjoyed eating during the holidays while maintaining my fasting schedule. We have a week off for Thanksgiving, so there was a LOT of eating at my house. My eldest son and his girlfriend stayed with us for a week during his college break. I was constantly cooking for others, whether it was breakfast waffles, scrumptious lunches, or hearty dinners. I never ate breakfast, but I did consume lunch and dinner every day.

Thanksgiving was also a significant food holiday. However, I counterbalanced the feasting days with days with shorter window times. The Monday following Thanksgiving, I felt extremely stuffed, but after a few days, I began to feel like myself again.

When I measured my waist on the 14th of December, I discovered that I had lost an inch since November 14th, when I had last measured. I was able to maintain a balance between feasting and fasting. Obviously, you should not forget about Christmas! If you're like me, the holiday is centred on food and parties. Parties are simple; they are typically visible from my window. Once my window is open, I can eat whatever I want without any remorse. The most difficult times are when food is constantly available, such as when sweets are constantly being produced. Early in December, students begin bringing me sweet treats as a teacher.

I've learned to save them until I get home, and if I'm hungry, I'll eat something in my window.

On occasion, you do wish to unwind and fully embrace the festivities. On the last day of school before Christmas break, I decided to do that. Students have a half-day, and there is always a luncheon for faculty and staff. I considered declining the luncheon but ultimately decided to embrace the day as the food festival that it could be. Honestly, I miss Chick-fil-breakfast A's the most during my fast. I am sorry if you are unfamiliar with that particular fast-food restaurant. This is a staple in the south. Their breakfast is only available during breakfast hours, Monday through Saturday, because they are closed on Sunday. That day, I chose to consume a chicken biscuit meal. And I would consume the sugary treats.

I would also consume lunch. I would then consume dinner that evening. Sigh. By 9:00 a.m., I already felt disgusting and was tired of eating.

You'll be relieved to hear that I persevered, and by the end of the day, I had eliminated feasting from my system entirely. Call the day a "metabolic boost" and move on. Occasionally, we require days like that to remind us why we choose to fast. The following day, I was completely prepared to resume my intermittent fasting regimen. It was actually a relief.

Feast, followed by a fast. I feel so much better when I practise intermittent fasting than when I eat continuously. Stunningly superior. I am certain that I will never return to my previous eating habits because they are so much better.

This one day of excess assisted me in staying somewhat on track on Christmas Eve and Christmas Day. I adhered to a 6-hour window on Christmas Eve and an 8-hour window on Christmas Day. I just didn't feel like overdoing it again. I ate whatever appeared appetising, but I closed my window before becoming bloated or miserable. Over the next few days, I naturally had little appetite. In fact, I was so busy on both days that I didn't open my window until after 6 p.m. It was nice to heed the message from my satiety hormones that I didn't need to eat much.

I decided to try on my honesty pants two days after Christmas. You understand what I mean; there are certain articles of clothing that do not stretch at all, and these items will never misrepresent your weight. I own two pairs of these pants, and I was able to put them on with ease and without a muffin top. I believe they were more comfortable than when I first tried them on in the fall.

I told you about my indulgences on cruises, during Thanksgiving, and at Christmas to demonstrate that I am not a perfect intermittent faster. Yes, intermittent fasting is my way of life. I adhere to it nearly every day. However, I make time to live my life when I determine it is worthwhile. On special occasions, such as vacations and life celebrations, you may choose to feast rather than fast. As long as intermittent fasting is a lifestyle choice, it is acceptable. Fasting is, after all, a lifestyle, not a religion.

Chapter 7: What is the One Meal Per Day Intermittent Fasting Diet?

In this chapter, we will examine OMAD in depth to determine if this intermittent fasting technique is right for you.

What is the OMAD diet exactly?

OMAD is an abbreviation for one meal per day.

If this acronym seems familiar, do not confuse it with GOMAD, which refers to the practise of consuming one gallon of milk per day in order to gain muscle.

OMAD is frequently utilised to reduce weight and improve body composition.

In comparison to the typical American diet of three meals and two snacks per day, the idea of consuming only one meal per day may seem excessive.

In contrast, eating less frequently has been the norm for the majority of human history.

From 2 million to 10,000 years ago, humans were apex predators, consuming enormous animals known as megafauna and then starving until the next successful hunt.

Only a few thousand years ago, fasting was still a common practise.

The Romans believed that consuming a single meal per day was healthier.

They werc preoccupied with digestion, and consuming multiple meals was deemed gluttonous.

This historical precedent continues to influence our genomes at present.

A number of adaptive responses are triggered by fasting: the brain thinks faster, blood vessels dilate, and muscles become more resistant to lactic acid.

45

From an evolutionary perspective, these traits make for excellent hunters.

It makes sense when you consider that those who hunted better when they were hungry survived and passed on their genes to us.

In contrast, failing to fast and consuming food constantly can make us fatter, slower, and less intelligent.

According to scientists, humans can thrive despite intermittent food shortages.

OMAD is an extreme variant of the intermittent fasting regimens that we have previously examined. This type of IF is also referred to as intermittent fasting because you consume all of your daily calories in a single meal.

OMAD requires daily fasting for approximately 23 hours. Within your one-hour eating window, you may eat as much as you wish. The majority of people prefer to eat at the same time each day.

Although the OMAD diet has gained popularity in part due to the belief that you can eat whatever you want and still lose weight, research demonstrates the importance of refuelling with wholesome whole meals.

Because fasting stimulates cellular renewal, this is the case. Feeding these young, ravenous cells high-carb processed garbage, which is prevalent in the Standard American Diet, can lead to malignant tumours and inflammation.

The majority of OMAD adherents prefer to eat around midday or at the end of the day, but not so late as to impede digestion before bedtime.

Because OMAD requires large meals, the timing of meals is crucial. Consider eating one meal per day after completing the majority of your daily activities.

You would not, for instance, consume a 3,000-calorie lunch and then immediately run or swim.

OMAD participants must also remember to eat enough.

The majority of people require at least 2,000 calories per day to thrive.

This may be difficult to consume in a single meal unless you consume high-energy foods such as steak or butter. Too few calories can harm the immune system, slow the thyroid, and make weight loss more challenging.

Likewise, individuals with a high calorie requirement should avoid OMAD fasting.

Superfoods such as salmon roe and oysters, as well as high-quality meat, eggs, and healthy fats, form the ideal foundation for an OMAD diet.

Supplements containing organ meat are an excellent way to ensure that you meet your micronutrient needs.

Chapter 8: Benefits Of Intermittent Fasting

The proper functioning of the human body and the metabolism, in particular, enables a greater sense of satisfaction and a healthier feeling. However, specialists describe intermittent fasting as a stimulant of metabolic and health functions. In fact, its benefits to the body are substantial. I can see why it would be interesting to incorporate it into our lifestyle. By fasting, you protect your body from numerous diseases. Let us now turn to the necessary explanations for a better grasp.

• QUICKLY CLEANS THE BODY

Numerous diseases are caused by the toxins and wastes produced by the human digestive system. The majority of these toxins come from our diet, especially when it is unhealthy. The human body must eliminate these toxins and maintain the highest quality biochemical components. Obviously, certain daily habits, such as drinking more water, continue to be necessary for the elimination of toxins. Sadly, the body does not always receive sufficient water to eliminate all of these toxins. A certain amount of water (between 1.5 and 2 litres) is necessary for the proper development of the body. In contrast, intermittent fasting activates the body's "cleansing" system.

• What exactly is homeostasis?

Without rest, the body is constantly digesting food. Under these circumstances, the body is incapable of mobilising the vital energy required to activate its "cleansing system." Even specialists are formal about this, as studies have demonstrated: Overeating inhibits the body's ability to heal itself. This is how numerous diseases develop. In contrast, when the body is temporarily deprived of food, its self-healing abilities are activated. The body's cleansing process begins. This stage is known as homeostasis.

• PERIODIC FASTING TO COMBAT DISEASES

By intermittently fasting, every individual protects himself from a variety of diseases. Intermittent fasting reduces the likelihood of cardiovascular disease. I now understand that a diet that is poorly adapted favours this type of disease. Conversely, intermittent fasting reduces the risk of diabetes and improves bad cholesterol levels. If you wish to reduce your blood cholesterol levels, you should not hesitate to engage in intermittent fasting.

• AN IDEAL WEIGHT

Whether you are a man or a woman, maintaining your weight requires you to eat according to your actual needs. Failure to comply with this rule will inevitably result in extra pounds. However, poor nutrition is not the only enemy of the ideal weight. In addition, there is a lack of physical activity or an exhausting or toxic mode. Intermittent fasting is therefore an ally in the pursuit of the ideal weight. Intermittent fasting is a safe method for managing body weight and satiety.

• WHEN DOES FASTING BECOME DANGEROUS?

The breakdown of the heart muscle, the myocardium, is particularly dangerous. Even with a certain amount of protein intake, rapid weight loss can result in a significant mobilisation of body protein from the myocardium. This is especially true for average-weight or slightly overweight individuals, who lose more fat-free body mass, i.e. muscle, during fasting than extremely obese individuals. Therefore, patients with existing heart disease should only fast under specific conditions and medical supervision.

• NUTRITIONAL EVALUATION

As a measure of weight reduction, fasting is not categorised. Therapeutic fasting can motivate a change in lifestyle. Positive fasting experiences can lead to a healthier lifestyle and dietary changes. However, a fasting cure cannot replace necessary medical treatment.

The term "purifying," which is frequently associated with therapeutic fasting, cannot be supported by science. There is no accumulation of cinders and deposition of metabolites in a healthy human body. Substances that cannot be utilised are eliminated via the intestines and kidneys when adequate fluid intake is present.

Fasting treatments should only be administered as an inpatient or under medical supervision following a thorough physical examination. It should be noted that fasting affects the efficacy of medication, and dosages should be altered accordingly. In any case, a contract with the doctor is required. On the one hand, health complications are only manageable.

Chapter 9: Intermittent Fasting And The Health Of Women

Intermittent fasting is a healthy lifestyle for everyone, but it is especially beneficial for women over 50 who have gone through menopause and wish to maintain their fitness and lose weight gained during "The Change."

Menopause occurs in two stages: perimenopause, when the body prepares for change, and menopause, when menstruation ceases. The next phase of life is called postmenopause.

Perimenopause, menopause, and postmenopause are all natural phases of a woman's life, but they represent profound emotional and physical changes.

Perimenopause

Perimenopause varies from one woman to the next. It typically lasts four years, but for some women it can last as little as a few months or as long as a decade. Some women may experience it as early as their late 30s, while others may not experience it until their 50s.

During perimenopause, it is still possible for a woman to become pregnant, but the likelihood of pregnancy decreases. This is because your ovaries produce less and less oestrogen, causing your periods to become irregular. The source of the sex hormones oestrogen, progesterone, and testosterone is a woman's ovaries. The female hormones oestrogen and progesterone regulate menstruation. The body prepares for menopause by producing progressively less oestrogen.

As a woman's oestrogen levels decrease, the balance between oestrogen and progesterone becomes unbalanced. This is the reason why many women experience mood swings.

In addition to mood swings and irregular periods, perimenopause symptoms include the following:

dryness that can affect vaginal health and make sex uncomfortable periods that are extra heavy or very light (spotting) more frequent urination or leaking changes in premenstrual syndrome for women with PMS hot flashes and night sweats insomnia or other sleep problems weight gain

Although there is no cure for perimenopause, there are treatments that can provide relief for women with particularly severe symptoms. And, as we will discuss, the IF lifestyle can have a substantial impact on your life.

Menopause and Postmenopause

A woman has officially entered menopause when she has not had a period for an entire year. For the majority of women, this occurs in their 50s.

At this point in your life, you enter the postmenopause.

75% of women will experience hot flashes during the day or night for a period of time after menopause. Nighttime hot flashes are commonly referred to as night sweats because they can cause you to perspire so heavily that you awaken in a pool of sweat.

Hot flashes are caused by hormonal fluctuations. During a hot flash, your face may flush, you may perspire, and you may experience vertigo or heart palpitations. After menopause, you may experience hot flashes several times per day for as long as a year or two. In extreme cases, they are more durable.

Due to hormonal changes, a woman's risk of cardiovascular disease may increase following menopause. Increased blood pressure may be a result of hot flashes. Changes in hormones also affect levels of the lipids cholesterol and triglycerides, which aid in cell repair and energy storage.

Osteoporosis, a reduction in bone density caused by low calcium levels in the body, is an additional consequence of menopause for many women. Osteoporosis heightens the risk of bone fractures.

Hormonal changes that affect your metabolism cause weight gain. Your body begins to store more energy and consume less. This means that you will use fewer calories during normal activities than you did previously, making it more difficult to burn off the excess energy that your body stores as fat. The majority of weight gain typically occurs around the waist (a change comparable to the difference between teenage and adult female bodies).

The increased amount of testosterone in the postmenopausal hormone balance may cause hair loss or thinning on the scalp, as well as an increase in facial hair.

Many women continue to experience vaginal dryness, find sex to be painful, and have a diminished desire for sexual activity.

There is some speculation that menopause affects memory, but it is unclear whether this is a result of menopause or simply ageing.

All of these changes, coupled with the fact that menopause signifies the end of the possibility of childbearing — one of the defining characteristics of a young woman — can result in depression or other mental health issues. However, all is not lost! Let's examine how IF can assist.

Arguments for IF

Women can take both prescription and over-the-counter medications to alleviate menopause symptoms. Included in this category are hormone replacement therapies (HRT), sleep aids, vaginal lubricants, and various nutritional supplements.

Dietary modifications are also recommended to alleviate symptoms such as hot flashes:

avoiding spicy foods, alcohol, and caffeine

abstain from smoking and other unhealthy practises

consuming more soybeans, chickpeas, grains, flax, beans, fruits, and vegetables

To reiterate, menopause is a natural occurrence. It is part of the process of ageing. In addition to menopausal-related changes, your body undergoes numerous aging-related changes.

As your immune system slows down, your body will also heal more slowly.

Even if you do not have osteoporosis, your bones will lose density and your muscles will become less flexible and strong. This is the reason why many elderly become shorter.

Your digestive system will undergo alterations. You may have difficulty digesting some formerly simple-to-digest foods (often cheese or spicy food).

You will experience urinary incontinence or urinary leakage.

Memory and cognitive abilities deteriorate.

Your vision and hearing will deteriorate, necessitating glasses (or new glasses) and possibly hearing aids.

Your teeth and gums become increasingly prone to infection and decay.

The largest organ of the body, the skin, becomes more fragile and less elastic.

You are likely to undergo sexual transitions.

● As your metabolism slows, gaining weight becomes easier.

There is no way to stop the ageing process. However, it is possible to take lifestyle measures that will help you remain as healthy as possible and reduce the effects of menopause and ageing.

Intermittent fasting comes into play here. Fasting has been discussed as both a religious practise and a type of diet. Both are valid. Intermittent fasting is a method for incorporating these healthy practises into one's lifestyle. At its core, intermittent fasting (IF) is a discipline that enables you to harness the powers of spirituality, health, and diet. It is a way of life that mitigates the effects of menopause and ageing, allowing you to remain as healthy as possible for as long as possible.

Here are some examples of evidence supporting the advantages of IF:

The website healthline lists ten effects of IF supported by scientific evidence (Gunnars, 2016). Among them are hormonal changes that result in decreased insulin and increased human growth hormone (HGH) levels, the stimulation of cellular repair processes, and the activation of genes.

weight loss due to increased metabolism and decreased caloric intake decreased blood sugar and insulin resistance decreased cardiovascular disease risk factors

According to a study of obese mice published in the journal Endocrinology, a type of intermittent fasting known as alternate day fasting (AF) led to significant weight loss and an increase in lean mass (Gotthardt et al., 2016).

Multiple studies indicate that IF can result in increased HGH levels (Mawer, 2019).

According to a clinical study published in The American Journal of Clinical Nutrition, AF led to weight loss and improved cardiovascular health by reducing cholesterol, triglyceride, and blood pressure levels (Varady et al., 2009).

According to a study of female mice published in the journal Mechanisms of Ageing and Development, mice fed intermittently (4 consecutive days every 2 weeks) lived about 30% longer than those fed daily (Sogawa & Kubo, 2000). According to multiple studies published in Ageing Research Reviews, IF promotes cellular repair functions throughout the body (Bagherniya et al., 2018).

Continue reading to learn more about the benefits of the IF lifestyle, particularly for women over the age of 50.

Parmesan Egg Toast with Tomatoes

This breakfast is quick to make and delicious. You can substitute grape tomatoes if you have them on hand. They provide a healthy dose of vitamin C to your meal.

• one teaspoon of olive oil
• ½ teaspoon chopped garlic (about 1 clove)
• 6 cherry tomatoes, quartered
• ½ teaspoon salt
• ¼ teaspoon freshly ground black pepper
• 2 large eggs
• 2 slices reduced-calorie whole wheat toast
• 1 tablespoon shredded Parmesan cheese

In a small skillet, heat the olive oil over medium heat. Add the garlic and tomatoes to the pan and sauté for 2 minutes, stirring often. Season with salt and pepper, then transfer to a plate to keep warm.

In the same skillet, fry the eggs for 2 minutes. Turnover and cook to the desired doneness (30 seconds for over easy, 1 minute for over medium, 2 minutes for over well).

Place 1 egg on each slice of toast, top with half the tomatoes, and sprinkle with half the Parmesan cheese.

Yields 2 servings.

Chapter 10: The Role Of Your Body's Hormones In Your Journey To Lose Weight

Your ability to lose weight may be significantly influenced by hormones, which are frequently associated with mood. Their secretion from various glands could be stimulated by a vast array of stimuli. For instance, when blood sugar levels increase, the pancreas produces insulin. Important hormones that influence weight loss will be discussed in this section.

Insulin is produced when blood glucose levels increase. Objective: reducing blood sugar

Insulin facilitates glucose entry into cells for energy production. Any excess will be transported to the liver, where insulin will stimulate glycogen production.

After eating, your blood sugar will increase. Insulin will be secreted as a result of the spike. This is both typical and important! However, daily overeating and mindless carbohydrate nibbling lead to more frequent blood sugar spikes and insulin secretion. Insulin's primary function is to induce storage, so its consistent presence in the bloodstream indicates that storage is occurring. If we continue along this path for long enough, we will develop insulin resistance. This suggests that insulin is no longer effective because our bodies have developed resistance to it. The pancreas must now secrete more insulin in an effort to reduce blood sugar levels. Due to the excessive amount of insulin in your bloodstream, your body will enter a state of storage and the liver will produce glycogen and fat more rapidly than usual.

When blood glucose levels fall, glucagon is produced. Increasing glucose levels is the objective. Glucagon stimulates the release of glucose from glycogen by the liver. Adipose tissue, also known as fat tissue, is stimulated by glucagon to release stored fat into circulation.

As can be seen, glucagon has the exact opposite effect of insulin. By having this rogue in your system, your body will be able to enter an energy-burning phase.

In addition to aiding in the absorption of fat-soluble vitamins such as A, D, K, and E, boosting cognitive function, constructing cell membranes, and regulating hormones, high-quality fats are the true anti-aging secret. Not to mention that it is the only macronutrient that does not trigger the release of the fat-storage hormone insulin.

Omega-3 fatty acids for hydration, B vitamins for collagen and elastin formation, and trace minerals for repair, protection, and 20 antioxidants.

Regeneration of cells is essential for healthy skin. Include leafy greens and fibre to encourage the growth of beneficial gut bacteria, as well as wild fish rich in omega-3 fatty acids, vitamin D, and B vitamins; sardines are my personal favourite.

When you think of anti-aging products, sunscreen and serums typically come to mind. In the realm of anti-aging, skincare is effective, but there is another crucial weapon in your arsenal. What and how you consume has a significant impact on the molecular maturation of your entire body. The Fab Four and intermittent fasting are both simple and effective ways to assist your body's natural anti-aging processes.

Many dietary recommendations emphasise the importance of eating small meals every three to four hours to maintain a healthy metabolism. Recent endocrine research indicates, however, that eating in this manner leads to fatigue, decreased fat-burning, and accelerated ageing.

The longer your body spends digesting, the less time it has for rejuvenating activities such as cellular repair, autophagy (the elimination of damaged cells), antioxidant production, cognitive maintenance, hormone balancing, and inflammation reduction. Intermittent fasting enhances the anti-aging effects of these processes.

Chapter 11: Weight Loss Through Intermittent Fasting

Intermittent fasting, which is supported by scientific evidence, is a tried-and-true method for quick weight loss results.

I grew up believing that skipping breakfast was unhealthy. After a long weekend without food, it was determined that, as long as you have access to water, living on a desert island would be healthier than consuming junk food on a regular basis.

Why is intermittent fasting so effective for weight loss and fat reduction?

It simply creates an environment in which the body can effectively burn fat. Fasting inhibits hormones that cause weight gain while stimulating hormones that promote fat loss.

Over the thousands of years of human evolution, food has not always been as readily available as it is now. There is no doubt that they did not consistently consume three meals and two snacks per day. In order to survive, the human body had to adapt to using its fat reserves as fuel until the next meal. Due to this, there were times when we had nothing to eat.

According to studies, intermittent fasting is a highly effective method for weight loss, reducing body fat, enhancing body composition, lowering blood pressure, and delaying the ageing process.

The key to intermittent fasting for achieving our goals is strategically employing it to dramatically increase our metabolism. This will increase your fat burning while maintaining your lean muscle mass. Even after a month of fasting, the results are quite striking. If you are attempting to lose weight, intermittent fasting's benefits may be ideal.

How to shed pounds with Intermittent Fasting

You can expect to lose between 2 and 10 pounds during the first week of intermittent fasting. During the first month of fasting, many women lose 10 to 15 pounds. As long as you consume a healthy, balanced diet the rest of the time, you can do this.

Your ability to lose weight will depend on how well you adhere to your diet, exercise, and fasting procedures. It is reasonable to anticipate a monthly weight loss of up to 20 pounds. It will be easier to lose weight if you have more weight to lose.

But if you eat poorly the rest of the time, intermittent fasting will not be very effective for weight loss.

To lose weight using intermittent fasting, your diet must adhere to the same guidelines.

Consume an abundance of protein and nutritious fats.

- Eliminate from your diet refined carbohydrates, vegetable oils, junk food, and processed foods.

- Get the majority of your carbs from leafy greens

To lose weight, you must also restrict your caloric intake. The average individual grossly underestimates their consumption. To monitor your calorie intake, you should not be required to record each meal in a journal. It will be helpful to record and measure the food you consume for at least a few days to gain a better understanding of the quantity of food you consume.

It is prudent to eat until you feel slightly full before stopping. The goal is to refrain from eating after 10 to 20 minutes. Your brain only realises you're full after eating the food you just consumed.

Some individuals have difficulty going 16 to 24 hours without eating.

Other health benefits are associated with intermittent fasting (without any major side effects).

Intermittent fasting may improve blood sugar regulation, reduce the risk of cardiovascular disease, and improve body composition, among other scientifically supported health benefits.

IF may reverse type 2 diabetes, reduce blood pressure, reduce the risk of

Alzheimer's disease, and reduce waist circumference.

Please note that this is not medical advice, and intermittent fasting may or may not alleviate the symptoms listed above. Consultation with a physician for diagnostic or therapeutic advice is always advised. If you've struggled with eating disorders, fasting is not your best option.

Fasting may resurrect past eating disorders in which intake was restricted. If you have experienced eating disorders, consult your doctor or psychologist for medically evaluated health information.

Human growth hormone (HGH) levels rise naturally during fasting. If you have more human growth hormone, you will expend more fat and muscle. It is possible to lose hormonal abdominal fat by first balancing your hormones.

The neurotransmitter norepinephrine will also be delivered to your fat cells by your nervous system. Therefore, they must digest fat in order to use it as fuel.

Since you will not consume many calories during fasting, you will immediately begin calorie restriction. This means that calorie restriction will not be necessary because weight loss will occur naturally.

In addition, you can anticipate keeping your muscle tone. According to studies, intermittent fasting results in significantly less muscle loss than calorie restriction.

Fasting has also been shown to improve gut health and repair any gut lining damage. The condition of your stomach has a significant impact on your entire fat-burning metabolism. It will be difficult to lose weight if your digestive health is poor. Fasting provides your stomach with a break, giving it more time to heal.

If you are diabetic, pregnant, or nursing, I would not recommend intermittent fasting without your physician's consent. You can have low blood sugar or inadequate nutrient intake.

Method of Fasting 4:3

The 24-hour fasting days protocol can be easily adhered to by dividing the week into four eating days and three non-consecutive fasting days.

This is the most effective way to use the 24-hour fast when I need to intensify my efforts while maintaining consistency.

The 4:3 fasting week is broken down as follows:

Monday: Day of Fasting

- Tuesday: Consume - Wednesday: Abstinence

- Thursday: Consume Food - Friday: Abstain

- Saturday: Eat - Sunday: Eat

As can be seen, the non-fasting days are dispersed throughout the week. These non-fasting days are necessary for long-term success. If not, you may quickly become exhausted. Obviously, this schedule can be altered to suit your needs.

Even while fasting, you should still consume something every day. However, your daily calorie intake should not exceed 500. Lunch typically consists of something light, such as soup.

For the average person attempting to lose weight through fasting, three 24-hour fasts per week will be more manageable. You will still have four days per week to eat on a more regular schedule.

This allows you to continue eating on the weekends despite dietary restrictions. Weekends are typically filled with social gatherings with friends and family, making fasting challenging.

Finding what works for you and sticking to it are the two most important steps. I am familiar with people who have attempted a continuous calorie restriction diet but abandoned it quickly due to its difficulty.

People who have experimented with intermittent fasting in a variety of ways have discovered that it is extremely effective, resulting in significant weight loss.

It can be difficult to fast, but staying busy is essential. Your fasting days will pass much more quickly if you do not waste time sitting around and watching cooking shows on YouTube.

Start with the 5:2 fasting plan if the 4:3 fasting plan proves to be too difficult. This occurs when five days without fasting are followed by two consecutive fasting days.

What foods and beverages may be consumed during a fast?

Unfortunately, when most people hear about intermittent fasting they immediately withdraw (or intermediate fasting). But the fact that fasting is the most natural method of weight loss explains why it is so effective.

Most individuals who attempt calorie restriction revert to binge eating quickly.

The "hunger pains" are too intense for them, therefore.

This issue is resolved by intermittent fasting, which entails abstaining from food for brief periods before resuming normal eating.

Water, coffee, tea, and other zero-calorie beverages may be consumed to satisfy hunger. Energy drinks with zero calories will also work, but you must be cautious because they contain artificial sweeteners. Even artificial sweeteners with zero calories can cause weight gain. Coffee will help you burn more fat during your fast because it speeds up your metabolism.

Chapter 12: Implications For Women Of Intermittent Fasting

The primary difference between men and women in relation to intermittent fasting appears to be the impact of this eating pattern on female hormones and daily life. Women who intermittently fast typically experience improved menstrual cycles. Due to their heightened sensitivity to the effects of caloric restriction, women are able to undergo these changes.

Below are discussed the potential benefits of intermittent fasting, followed by the specifics of intermittent fasting for women, and then some Tips on Periodic Fasting.

Having confidence in one's own abilities is essential for achieving one's goals.

If you are interested in the health benefits of intermittent fasting, you must learn a great deal about it. Let's investigate this topic further.

Shedding The Pounds

Regularly fasting for shorter durations has been shown to reduce total energy expenditure, suggesting that it may be an effective and simple method of weight loss for women.

When it comes to preserving muscle mass in women over the age of 50, it appears that intermittent fasting is superior to continuous calorie restriction. This is especially crucial after menopause, when it becomes increasingly difficult to maintain muscle mass.

Benefits of Intermittent Fasting for Diabetes Management and Prevention in Both Men and Women Insulin levels and insulin resistance must be reduced in order to achieve this objective.

Slow Aging

According to scientific research on anti-aging effects, intermittent fasting may reduce key inflammatory markers. There is evidence that inflammation contributes to the ageing process, including skin pigmentation and metabolic alterations. Intermittent fasting may slow the ageing process by reducing age-related DNA degradation and accelerating DNA repair.

Due to its effects on hormone production, fasting has direct consequences for the thyroid. Certain studies have linked fasting to decreased levels of the hormone T3. It has been shown that intermittent fasting reduces hypothyroidism symptoms by influencing energy expenditure. Several women have also reported an increase in the effectiveness of their hypothyroidism medication and a decrease in inflammation.

Menopause is the natural and inevitable decline in sex hormones that occurs between the ages of 40 and 50 in women. Because the ovaries have stopped producing oestrogen and progesterone, menstruation ceases. Once a woman has gone a full year without having her period, she is considered to have entered menopause. However, amenorrhea is not the only menopause symptom (loss of periods).

Menopause can cause a number of unpleasant symptoms, including but not limited to: hot flashes, vaginal dryness, decreased libido, anxiety, sadness, an increased risk of heart disease, chills, nocturnal sweats, and mood swings. In addition to these unpleasant side effects, the menopause also causes significant metabolic changes. The decline in oestrogen and progesterone levels that occurs during menopause is a major factor in the metabolic sluggishness that occurs during this time. Often, women gain weight rapidly due to fluctuating hormone levels.

It has been shown that intermittent fasting can alleviate some of the symptoms of menopause. Intermittent fasting can alleviate menopausal symptoms including weight gain, insulin resistance, and sleep disruptions.

More Health Benefits

Animal and human studies have hinted at the possible health benefits of intermittent fasting.

Some studies have linked intermittent fasting to decreased levels of inflammatory markers. Persistent inflammation can result in weight gain and a variety of other health issues.

• Obese individuals who had practised intermittent fasting for weeks experienced a significant reduction in depressive symptoms and binge eating, as well as an improvement in body image.

• The practise of intermittent fasting can increase rodent lifespan by 33 to 83% (mice and rats). It is currently unknown whether and how this increases human lifespan.

• Intermittent fasting is more effective than constant calorie restriction at preserving muscle mass. Muscle increases the amount of energy expended at rest.

The importance of staying hydrated increases as one becomes accustomed to going long periods without eating. If you're hungry and want to try something natural, dilute some apple cider vinegar with water. This can aid in appetite suppression and weight loss.

When you're ready, ladies, proceed slowly and deliberately. See how your body reacts if you go without food for a few hours. You can then gradually increase your fasting intervals until you are skipping two meals simultaneously. After the fasting periods have ended, it is time to resume a healthy diet.

Chapter 13: Two Days Of Weekly Abstinence Is Recommended.

The 52-day intermittent fasting schedule, also known as the 5:2 diet, requires that you consume 20% of your normal daily caloric intake on the other two days of the week.

During fasting days, women should consume 500 calories and men should consume 600. If you choose to follow this plan, load up on calories the day before your fast to avoid overeating when it's time to break your fast.

Typically, fasting days are separated throughout the week. For instance, they might observe a fast on Mondays and Thursdays while eating normally on

95

other days. At least one non-fasting day should intervene between fasting days.

Every minute you're alive, you burn calories, even when you're sleeping. During sleep, your body uses glycogen stored in the liver to maintain stable blood sugar levels.

As a result, according to White, your body is accustomed to the fasting mechanisms.

"Your body is designed to compensate when it is deprived of food," she continues. The purpose of something like a fast is to extend the amount of time you rely on your internal fuel reserve.

In a small study, Trusted Source examined the effects of this type of fasting on 23 overweight women. In a single menstrual cycle, the women lost

4.8% of their body weight and 8.0% of their total body fat.

However, after five days of eating normally, the majority of women's measurements returned to normal.

What are economical genes?

How did our ancestors survive when the prey eluded them or the crops failed? Those who could store body fat to measure off in their spare time survived, whereas those who could not decomposed. This evolutionary adaptation explains why the vast majority of ultramodern humans, approximately 85 individuals, possess so-called frugal genes, which help us conserve energy and store fat. Moment, these thrifty genes are a curse rather than a blessing. Not only is food available nearly around-the-clock, but we do not even need to hunt or gather it!

Individuals with a strong hereditary predisposition to rotundity may not be suitable candidates for weight loss using conventional diet and exercise methods. In fact, if they decrease, they're

less likely to handle the load reduction. For people with a veritably strong inheritable predilection, sheer restraint is ineffective in neutralising their tendency to be fat. Typically, these individuals can only maintain weight loss under the supervision of a crocodile. They are also the most likely to interact with weight-loss medications or surgical procedures. Since the 1970s, the prevalence of rotundity among adults in the United States has been on the rise.

It is inconceivable that genes alone could explain such a rapid increase. Although the inheritable predilection to be fat varies extensively from person to person, the increase in body mass indicator appears to be nearly universal, cutting across all demographic groups. These findings highlight the significance of changes in our terrain that contribute to the obesity epidemic.

The exercise equation

The government currently recommends one hour of moderate to vigorous physical activity per day. But fewer than 25 percent of Americans meet this requirement. Our daily lives provide few opportunities for physical exertion. Due to frequent cuts to physical education classes, school-aged children exercise less frequently than they should. Numerous people drive to work and spend important of the day sitting at a computer outstation. We struggle to find time to visit a spa, play a sport, or engage in other forms of exercise due to our long work hours.

We drive to one-stop megastores, where we park close to the entrance, wheel our purchases on a shopping waggon, and then drive back home. The widespread use of vacuum cleaners, dishwashers, splint boasters, and a plethora of other appliances removes nearly all physical effort from daily tasks and may be one of the causes of obesity.

Chapter 14: What Supplements Should Be Taken During A Fast?

Some dietary supplements can interfere with fasting, while others can be consumed during fasting periods. Likewise, supplements support fasting. Regarding fasting, dietary supplements appear to be a confusing grey area. So, are supplements important? Typically, breaking the fast involves high-calorie foods and beverages. Therefore, nutritional supplements that stimulate digestion or increase insulin levels can also be included. It is essential to exercise caution when refilling inside. Other supplements should not be taken on an empty stomach, but they will not necessarily break the fast.

This dietary supplement, L-tyrosine, should be taken on an empty stomach, so it is acceptable to take it on an empty stomach. Although tyrosine is an amino acid, it is typically taken as a dietary supplement in low doses, so fasting is rarely interrupted.

These are beneficial gut bacteria, or probiotics. If your stomach acid levels are low, you should take certain probiotic supplements between meals. However, some are more effective when consumed with food. Therefore, it is essential to verify

label of your probiotic supplement for recommendations from the manufacturer. The majority of probiotics are calorie-free and should not hinder fasting.

Prebiotics should not be confused with probiotics, which are beneficial bacteria. Prebiotics are fibres that nourish gut bacteria to promote a healthy microbiome in the gut. However, it is not absorbed and does not stimulate insulin production. You must exercise caution.

Typically, electrolytes refer to potassium, sodium, magnesium, and calcium. It is acceptable to consume electrolyte supplements while fasting so long as they do not contain added sugars or calories. In fact, electrolytes can also aid in the management of the side effects associated with entering ketosis. Electrolytes also aid in hydration because they help the body retain water.

Assuming it is a pure creatine supplement and not one that has been sweetened, creatine has zero calories and does not affect insulin levels, so it will likely not break your fast.

What water-soluble vitamins Vitamins B and C do not require fat for absorption, so they can be taken during fasting with only water.

Vitamin C is typically well tolerated on an empty stomach, whereas vitamin B complexes can induce nausea when taken on an empty stomach. It can be processed or taken during a non-fasting period if necessary.

What is Intermittent Fasting (IF)? What is intermittent fasting specifically about? Almost everyone is familiar with the term fasting. The motives for fasting vary from one tribe to the next. Others sacrifice food to devote themselves to prayer, as part of a religious ceremony. Others lack food due to a lack of cause. In ancient societies, people worked in the fields and only ate when they rested. Intermittent fasting is not one of the fasting methods described previously. It is a choice and not a religious practise or one motivated by a lack of time or food. It is best described as an eating pattern consisting of alternating periods of eating and fasting, with each period lasting a specified amount of time. For instance, the 16:8 technique consists of a 16-hour fasting period and an 8-hour eating period. Please note that this is not a diet, but rather an eating habit.

Less emphasis is placed on the meals you should consume, and more on when you should consume them. Does this mean you can consume whatever you desire? No, unfortunately. As with all other aspects of life, you will receive what you invest. Eating healthfully is one of the three pillars of fat-burning success. Does this mean you must subsist solely on chicken and broccoli? No, obviously not.

As humans, I believe in enjoying life, but as you well know, moderation is essential. It is essential to note that intermittent fasting is not a fad diet that will be popular for a short time and then fade away like other weight loss programmes. Even if you are just learning about it now, it has existed for a very long time and has been popular for many years (even if you are learning about it just now). It is currently one of the most popular health and fitness trends in the world. Numerous health and fitness professionals endorse it.

HOW FAT IS STORED & BURNT
Intermittent fasting has been tried and proven to be an effective fat-burning and weight-loss method. But how exactly does it operate? Before examining how something works, it is essential to understand two crucial factors:

The manner in which the body stores energy

How the body makes use of energy

The body is either in a state of energy storage or energy expenditure. There exists no middle ground. What does this signifier? If you are not burning glucose (sugar), you are essentially storing it as glycogen or fat. Does this imply that you must consistently exercise? The short answer is no. In reality, exercise only accounts for 10% to 15% of the equation for weight loss (more on this later) (more about that later). Your body expends energy in numerous ways. Even when you are immobile and doing nothing, your body expends energy to perform essential life functions.

Nevertheless, even if your cells are consuming glucose and expending energy, any surplus will be stored. This qualifies as a storage condition. Wait! If we either store or burn sugar, logic dictates that consuming fewer calories and engaging in more physical activity should result in weight loss. It seems straightforward, correct? Obviously, if you're reading this, you've tried this strategy without success. Either you saw initial results that quickly evaporated or you regained all the weight when you returned to your normal lifestyle. Then, how can I lose weight? To gain a better perspective, we must comprehend two principles:

How glucose (sugar) is stored and burned for energy, or utilised.

The role of our hormones in this process

How does energy storage occur?
The body can use both glycogen and fat to store energy. As a result of digestion, food (yum) is broken down into a variety of macronutrients. These macronutrients are ingested by the body, absorbed into the bloodstream, and transported to our cells, where they serve a variety of functions. Carbohydrates, for instance, are

converted to glucose (sugar), which is then absorbed by the bloodstream and transported to the cells, where it is utilised for energy.

Conversely, if there is an excess of glucose in the blood (hyperglycemia), it will be stored as glycogen through a process known as glycogenesis. The body's glycogen storage capacity is maximal.

Once these reserves are depleted, any excess glucose is converted into fat through a process called lipogenesis.

How is energy utilised?
When our cells require more energy than the blood can provide, glycogen is converted back into glucose via a process known as glycolysis (low blood sugar). To restore normal blood sugar levels, glycogen reserves are depleted

gradually. As soon as these reserves are depleted, the lipolysis process, which breaks down fat for energy, will begin.

Chapter 15: Detailed Instructions For Planning An Efficient Fast

You can take steps to prepare your body for the sudden, extreme change in diet that will occur during a fast. These are the steps to consider when attempting to resume a fast pace.

1 Consult your primary care physician or medical provider prior to fasting. There are numerous obvious motivations to fast, regardless of whether you have a disease. However, there are potential health risks with fasting, which you should discuss with an authorised expert before diving into the deep end of fasting.

Due to changes in your blood science, a few medications you take may pose a risk to your health during fasting.

Fasting may not be ideal for people with medical issues, such as pregnancy, severe disease, low pulse, and that's just the tip of the iceberg. Prior to fasting, you should consult with your primary care physician if you have any illness.

Your primary care doctor may order a urine or blood test prior to the fasting period.

2 Determine the type and duration of fasting you will practise. There are numerous fasting practises. Some include simply drinking water, others include drinking juices (or clear fluids), and others are for extraterrestrial reasons, weight loss, or to treat a disease. You must determine which option is most suitable for you. Water fasting is a more rigorous form of fasting and one of the more difficult types. You can do it anywhere between 1 and 40 days (though 40 days is pushing it and is not recommended without a specialist's approval). Water fasting can be hazardous to your health both while you

are fasting and after you have completed the fast. You must begin and conclude a multi-day juice diet. The juice fast is one of the safer bets for fasting, since you're actually receiving nutrients from the juices you're drinking; therefore, it is less rigorous than the water fast and is recommended. 1 to 10 days is the typical duration of a juice fast. You must consume only vegetable and organic product juices, as well as homegrown teas and vegetable stock.

The Expert Scrub is a quick drink that combines the water quick and the juice quick. For approximately ten days, you consume freshly crushed lemons, water, and maple syrup. This is a more convenient fast because you will still receive some calories (albeit not however numerous as you seem to be utilised to).

Fasting periods can last between 1 and 40 days, contingent upon your objective and the type of quick you're doing (juice quick, water quick, clear fluid quick, etc.), as this will determine how your body adjusts to having the vast majority of its calories removed.

Prepare yourself for the changes that may occur in your body. Fasting is associated with eliminating the toxins that have accumulated in your body (it will do this regardless of whether you're fasting for religious or spiritual reasons), so you should be prepared to feel ill and weak, particularly in the beginning.

As a result of the interaction between fasting and detoxification, fasting may result in side effects such as diarrhoea, fatigue and weakness, increased personal odour, headaches, and more.

Consider taking a break from work or relaxing more throughout the day to accommodate the effects of fasting on your body.

Reduce your consumption of all ongoing and drugs 1 to approximately fourteen days before fasting The more trash you eliminate from your diet, the easier the fast will be on you and your body. Stop drinking alcohol gradually and attempt to eliminate or quit smoking entirely. [5] This strategy will reduce any potential withdrawal symptoms you may experience during the fasting process, as well as reduce the amount of toxins in your body that the fast will work to eliminate. Included in addictive substances and substances are alcoholic beverages, carbonated beverages such as coffee, tea, and pop, and cigarettes or cigars.

Adjust your diet approximately one to fourteen days prior to fasting. Similar to quitting drugs, you will need to alter your diet so that you can adhere to the fast more easily.

Eliminating a few things per day is an effective method for slipping into this state (refined sugar items in the several days, meat in the following couple, and afterward dairy, and so on.).

Reduce your consumption of chocolate and other foods that are high in refined sugar and fat, such as soft drinks, chocolate, treats, and prepared foods.

[6] Consume dinners in smaller portions, so your digestive system doesn't have to work as hard to fill up, and your body becomes accustomed to operating on fewer calories than it normally does.

Reduce your intake of meats and dairy products.

Consume fragments of cooked or raw leafy foods.

Reduce your caloric intake one to two days prior to fasting. This is the point at which you must truly ensure that your body is prepared, and consequently, individuals cannot simply jump into a fast without prior preparation (or on the other hand in the event that they do, they have a lot harder time during the actual quick).

Consume a lot of fluids. Juices made from fresh, unprocessed fruits and vegetables to rehydrate leafy foods. You will need to increase your fluid intake during the pre-fast in order to keep your body hydrated and prepare it for a period of time without food.

7. Engage in moderate exercise. You would prefer not to engage in an excessive amount of activity, but you must engage in some to keep the lymphatic fluid moving and the vascular system healthy. Perform some slow yoga or go for a moderate walk. Know that you will feel exhausted, even on the pre-quick eating routine, but don't worry about it. Simply modify your typical levels of activity to accommodate the

sluggishness. Get plenty of rest. Whether you get sufficient rest and sleep will determine how well you perform on the fast and how quickly you recover afterwards. Ensure that you are getting adequate rest in the evening and that you are relaxing throughout the day. Therefore, it is preferable to prepare for a quick, as opposed to rushing in carelessly. You'll require time to recuperate

www.ingramcontent.com/pod-product-compliance
Lightning Source LLC
Chambersburg PA
CBHW060948050426
42337CB00052B/1940